I

G000149870

15 Ways to
S
Bladder Inflammation Using Imagery

Imagery has a profound physiological effect on IC patients, influencing the body's systems: immune, endocrine, nervous, cardiovascular, respiratory and gastro-intestinal.

When you have a positive outlook, use your imagination and have positive self-talk, the body's chemistry changes by turning up the feel-good chemicals, allowing stress and the IC symptoms to be better managed.

- Imagination is humanity's oldest healing method.
- Imagination changes the body's chemistry.
- Imagine Interstitial Cystitis (IC) leaving your body.

Pick up this Amazing Itty Bitty Interstitial Cystitis (IC) book and share it with your doctors and friends.

Your Amazing Itty Bitty® Interstitial Cystitis (IC) Book

15 Ways to Address Bladder Inflammation Using Imagery

Rhona Jordan
C.GIt., C.CHt.

Acknowledgments

Jamie Taylor, DPT, *was the first to invite me to use imagery with her pelvic floor PT patients. Jamie, thank you for having the vision and trust in imagery. Your faith in this work changed my life path and entire career.*

Gail Wetzler, DPT, *a leader and innovator for women's health, helped my body when it needed her most and I am forever grateful.*

Robin Christenson, DPT, *created Womanology and Restore Him Physical Therapy, one of the first women's health clinics in Orange County, California. Robin generously invited me to use imagery with her patients. Thank you for your support.*

Julie Sarton, DPT *is the owner of Sarton Physical Therapy, where I have imagined with her patients for years. Julie, thank you for your trust, insight, wisdom and true contagious, loving spirit.*

Ruth Velicki, DPT. *I met Ruth when we were both speaking at a conference. Ruth had suffered with IC for years and one of the gifts the illness gave her was to become a powerful healer and teacher. Thank you for your friendship and generously sharing your remarkable story.*

Stop by our Itty Bitty® website to find more information about IC and Imagery at:

www.ittybittypublishing.com

Or visit Rhona Jordan at

www.RhonaImagery.com

Table of Contents

Introduction

My heart goes out to those who experience interstitial cystitis (IC). As a Certified Imagery Therapist, I have been working with IC patients for over ten years and have seen the benefits of imagery in many different phases of IC treatment. Most of the female and male patients I work with share these universal experiences and fears:

- Loss of identity, wanting their life back.
- Flare-ups causing cancellation of important life events.
- Increasing and referred pain.
- Pain during and after sex.
- Feeling overwhelmed by unending doctor visits, medical tests, prescriptions, procedures, instillations, injections or surgery.
- Fear of the bladder never healing.
- Feeling alone and isolated, not understood by family, friends and most doctors.
- Drastic lifestyle changes including the urgency to find a public bathroom and eliminating foods and drinks from their diet.
- Handling the stress of IC, along with the stress of everything else.

The IC Journey

With multiple holistic approaches, combinations of treatments, prescriptions, procedures, therapies and diet alterations, you can take control of your body and your life and manage, heal and create a more comfortable new normal.

Let's begin with better understanding of imagery for managing and healing interstitial cystitis (IC). Imagery is the oldest form of healing on the planet; we have always used our imagination. Whatever we are thinking or imagining releases the corresponding chemicals in the body. We know that chronic pain can rewire the brain to expect more pain. Biology changes with self/internal dialog.

Example: When you have a positive experience, the body releases feel-good chemicals: serotonin, endorphins, oxytocin and dopamine. And when you have a painful experience, the body produces cortisol and adrenalin. A little cortisol and adrenalin are good, however, big doses daily compromise the immune system and even take our thinking offline. It is never easy to make good decisions when experiencing stress, fear, anger or pain, however – *imagery is the chemical game changer!* With positive imagery, our self-dialog changes and this allows for self-nurturing, encouragement, hope, peace and acceptance. Positive imagery supports the body's powerful healing ability, hence, its direct impact on treating IC.

IC Imagery 1
Morning Stretch
Stretching, Exercise and Moving the Body

Stretching is essential to elongate the pelvic floor muscles and make them stronger.

1. The body wants to feel strong, limber and flexible.
2. Know that you are taking ACTION toward healing and a new normal.
3. Plan a time every day to stretch for a few minutes.
4. It is best to stretch both in the morning and in the evening. The morning stretch exercise can be found on the following page and the evening stretch is covered in IC Imagery 2, *Evening Stretch*.

Morning Stretch to Awaken

- Imagine the morning Sun rising from the East as you salute another new day in which to walk this beautiful earth.
- Face the East and stretch your arms and body toward the Sun.
- Follow the movements of the Sun with your body as you stretch.
- Imagine the Sun rising and moving across the horizon until it sets in the West.
- Breathe oxygen deeply into your cells, molecules, tissues and muscles, sending it wherever your body is calling out for attention.
- Imagine acknowledging the body, as you release the breath.
- Imagine blowing out and away the discomfort.
- Imagine you are breathing in peace and hope.
- Imagine increasing flexibility in the mind's awareness.
- Imagine releasing fatigue and inviting your body to feel energized and flexible.
- Talk to your body; thank it for doing the best it can today.

IC Imagery 2
Evening Stretch
Sleep is a State of Consciousness

There are two sleep states. When you are in deep sleep there is little awareness. But when you are in the dream state, your consciousness is focused inward and you experience a world behind closed eyes: activities, buildings, people, conversations, travel, weather, emotions and actions; in short, a different view of the universe inside of you.

1. Chinese medicine teaches that when you are asleep, the body uses that time to focus on each organ for healing and rejuvenation.
2. Sleep is one of the most important factors in maintaining mental, emotional and physical health.
3. Restful sleep supports the immune system and the ability to think clearly, allowing you to make good decisions.
4. The moon represents femininity, the menstrual cycle and knowingness or woman's natural intuition.
5. Women are intuitively connected to the moon with her magnetic forces influencing the tides of the sea and the fluid tides in the body.

Evening Stretch to Sleep

- Imagine connecting with the powerful and beautiful moon.
- Imagine the moon's beauty and softness.
- Imagine the moon's strong magnetic pull.
- Imagine stretching and reaching for the beautiful full moon, as if it were a ball.
- Hold the moon until you set the moon down below the horizon.
- Tighten and release the muscles used during the day: arms, back, torso and legs.
- Imagine giving yourself permission to let your body rest, regenerate, heal, sleep and dream.
- Imagine releasing melatonin, your own natural sleep chemical.
- Smell your pillow case and know that you are safe and that you can sleep peacefully with the moon above.
- Imagine that if you should awaken during the night, you are able to return quickly to sleep and wake up at the appropriate hour the next morning.

IC Imagery 3
Relaxing Bath

This relaxing bath imagery helps to lessen IC symptoms by releasing tension and tightness in the stomach, bladder and pelvic floor.

1. Stretch your arm, torso and legs, while taking a few deep breaths to settle down.
2. Give your body permission to rest and relax in the comfort of the warm water.
3. Have a mental conversation with your body, loving the self unconditionally right now just as it is.
4. Perhaps light a candle or turn on music to set the mood and step into the warm bath.
5. Allow the warm waters to enfold and wrap around your body, relaxing the pelvic floor muscles that hold the bladder in place.
6. Perhaps close your eyes and feel your body floating, peaceful and quiet.
7. This is your sacred time to meditate or just be and rest.

Images for Your Relaxing Bath

- Imagine releasing any tensions or discomfort.
- Imagine the bladder floating.
- Imagine calming the nerve endings, cooling the urethra, bladder and the bladder lining.
- Imagine your body is listening to your every healing thought and responding to its own intuitive wisdom.
- Imagine spending some time here enjoying "no sense of gravity" – peaceful, quiet, simply floating.
- Imagine the discomfort being washed away when you empty the bathtub.
- Let go of the outcome and experience being fully here in this moment.

IC Imagery 4
Urgency
Acknowledging the Body's Response

The urgency you feel is the body trying frequently to clean itself by pressure-flushing the urine from the bladder.

1. When you become angry at the urgency and inconvenience, that strong emotion alters the chemical healing response and creates cortisol and adrenalin in the body.
2. The urgency is temporary, not forever.
3. The body naturally wants to be well.
4. As you learn about the many ways to support your healing, the body responds accordingly.
5. The mind is always eavesdropping on our thoughts and feelings.
6. Things to tell the body: the bladder is safe, loved and healing.

Images for Your Sense of Urgency

- Imagine while urinating that the bladder is completely emptying itself.
- Imagine that as the bladder is completely emptying itself of urine, it is also releasing the discomfort.
- Imagine as the bladder re-fills, the lining is soothed, cooled and remembers wellness.
- Imagine the bladder and the bladder lining using the body's inner pharmacy and releasing the body's natural morphine.
- Imagine you can feel the healing, cooling and soothing.
- Imagine the pelvic floor muscles relaxed and calm.
- Imagine the nervous system calm and balanced with the other body systems.

IC Imagery 5
Feeling Overwhelmed and the Importance of Loving Self

We all need to share love and to be loved. Love is the greatest healer because it changes the chemistry in our body. Loving yourself unconditionally is the most important emotion for healing any condition in the body.

1. When the body releases the feel-good hormones, serotonin and oxytocin, the immune system is naturally affected.
2. Love is the key here for change and healing.
3. When someone first falls in love, they hardly ever even get a cold.
4. Love yourself.
5. Be well.

Images for Loving Yourself

- Imagine love meeting all your essential needs.
- Imagine supporting your powerful immune system by having healthy relationships with family, friends and co-workers, the clerk at the store, the medical staff.
- Imagine taking it one step at a time and not running the whole 10K marathon in three minutes.
- Imagine you as a spiritual being and engage in your spirituality.
- Imagine a creative lifestyle for the new normal that is uplifting.
- Imagine choosing how to spend each day in activity, optimism and happiness.
- Imagine letting go of the illusions of the fear-based thought forms, including all the "what ifs" that do not serve you on any level.
- Imagine no longer telling the old story of your pain and telling the new story of the body's healing abilities.

IC Imagery 6
Push Through the Challenge
with Gratitude
You were Born and
You are Walking on this Earth.
You are a Miracle

Celebrate! You are breathing and here on this beautiful earth.

1. Gratitude is a thought that changes the chemistry in the body, enhancing the immune system and clear thinking.
2. The opposite is fear, also a thought form.
3. If you have a fearful thought, you can change it.
4. Every moment of your existence, you are offered opportunities.
5. Every thought, word and action can become a self-fulfilled prophecy.
6. Choice: Experience the day in positivity or negativity.
7. Choice: The words you say to yourself and the words you say to others.
8. Choice: Embrace the unknown and live in the moment.

Gratitude

- Be grateful you have feet as you walk with each step to the bathroom.
- Be grateful for your existence.
- Be grateful for expanded awareness, knowledge and wisdom.
- Be grateful for the healing ability within your body.
- Be grateful for the inner voice of guidance.

Additional Images

- Imagine enlightenment and awaken your flexible mind.
- Imagine awakening your intuition.
- Imagine balance with your thoughts and actions.
- Imagine hope and happiness in each action.
- Imagine strength, courage, focused attention on well-being.
- Imagine being in the state of pure potential.
- Imagine you are expanded awareness in the ever-expanding universe.
- Imagine your full expression of unconditional love for self and for others.

IC Imagery 7
Eliminating Some Foods and Drinks

It is important to add a Nutritionist to your health advisor team. Some foods are particularly helpful, while other foods are irritating.

1. Cooked food is easier to digest.
2. Avoid constipation, as it increases pressure on the bladder and straining can cause other challenges.
3. A few foods tend to aggravate and increase discomfort.
4. Tannins: Avoid acidic foods, most citrus fruits and fruit drinks and wines that contain tannins.
5. Caffeine and acidic teas are diuretic.
6. Avoid spicy foods.
7. Avoid carbonated / bubbled beverages.
8. Avoid foods containing yeast such as cake, white bread, candy and rice.
9. Fried foods clog arteries and could restrict blood flow to the pelvic floor.
10. Acidic foods, with the addition of stress and worry, create higher cortisol levels compromising the adrenal glands and immune system, decrease blood flow to the bowel and affect the alkalizing oxygen system for the bladder.

What to Do About Food and Drink

There are wonderful books for you to read that offer many delicious food choices with healing alkaline recipes for IC management. For the greatest benefit, use these images to compliment your new nutrition plan.

- Imagine your body is a natural pharmacy for healing.
- Imagine the food as healing and working with your body's pharmacy.
- Imagine enjoying your food choices for comfort.
- Imagine the foods that enter your body are soothing.
- Imagine the body in balance with acidity and alkalinity.

IC Imagery 8
Meditation
Your Higher Self Wants You to Make Choices Creating Peace, Health, Love and Meaning in Your Life

Meditation is not a religion; it is a practice that takes our awareness to the level of our spirit, which is the same spirit that connects everything in creation. The benefits of meditation are endless; here are just a few:

1. Reduces stress and overreaction.
2. Opens the desire to be creative.
3. Improves decision-making.
4. Increases level of intelligence.
5. Supports a healthy immune system.
6. Enhances brain matter.
7. Calms blood pressure.
8. Supports a more loving, kind and gentle personality.
9. Expands awareness and intuition.
10. Meditation benefits are accumulative in the body and mind.
11. Meditate daily whenever you are able from 1 minute to 30 minutes.
12. Be easy on yourself.
13. The mind and body are inseparable.

Meditation Exercise

- Sit upright and comfortably.
- Settle into your body, aware of all the sounds around you, aware of your natural breathing and allow yourself to just be still.
- Close your eyes so you can go within and simply allow yourself this precious time.
- When your thoughts come, acknowledge them, let them go.
- This simple intention and action is profound for your body and mind.
- Be present in the moment.

IC Imagery 9
The New Normal During the
Process of Healing IC
Using Your Knowledge

The new normal means doing some things differently for a while, such as doing only what you can and getting plenty of rest.

1. Trust yourself and trust your body's healing abilities. You will get through this.
2. You are stronger than you think.
3. You are effective in relieving symptoms.
4. You are able to increase your functional abilities.
5. You have tolerance and compassion for your body.
6. You can calm and balance your body's entire system.
7. You will return to bible study or playing with the children.
8. You are more powerful than you think you are.

Images for the New Normal

Thoughts are powerful. Thoughts support the immune, endocrine and nervous systems. A vivid or erotic thought causes powerful changes in the body: all the systems, including pelvic floor, cardiovascular, respiratory and gastrointestinal are involved. Here are some images for this healing process:

- Imagine yourself being the best you can be as you are healing.
- Imagine today is better than yesterday and tomorrow will be even better.
- Imagine allowing the bladder, urethra, pelvic floor to feel calm, safe, soothed and relaxed.
- Imagine using all the knowledge you are gathering to heal your IC.

Here are additional ways in which you can put your healing thoughts into action:

- Be aware of your choices and actions with every thought.
- Laugh every day, even if you need to rent a funny movie.
- Be very mindful of the self-talk, the self-fulfilling prophecy.
- Help someone else feel better about their experiences.

IC Imagery 10
Worry and Fear
Scientists Proved Worry and Fearful Thoughts Create a Wave Pattern that Turns into Self-fulfilling Prophesies

Have you ever considered what happens to your physical body when you worry? Perhaps you have heard someone say:

"I am worried sick."

"I am so worried that I could just die."

"I am so worried that I can't think."

During the IC journey, you are offered many experiences and many different opportunities to learn about the journey. Fear and worry undermine these possibilities.

1. Worry is a thought form based on fear about the past or the future and not about living in the present.
2. Reaction to worry changes the body chemistry, compromising the immune system.
3. Worry fogs our ability to think clearly, taking the mind offline.
4. Worry affects the immune system and prevents you from getting well sooner.
5. You tell yourself a worrisome, fearful story, believe it and then make that story true for you; a self-fulfilling prophecy.

Images to Overcome Fear and Worry

- Imagine you are able to fully embrace the unknown – and trust the process.
- Imagine the thought forms based on fear or worry are exchanged for confidence and courage.
- Imagine most thoughts are positive.

IC Imagery 11
Mindfulness and IC
Being Aware, Being Present with Self, The Universe, the Earth and All Beings

Mindfulness is being totally awake, aware and conscious of your choices, words, actions and consequences, with no judgments.

1. Mindfulness is the witness.
2. Mindfulness is no judgment.
3. Mindfulness is the now.
4. Mindfulness is the wonder of creation.
5. Mindfulness is feeling the rain on your skin.
6. Mindfulness is feeling the breath enter and then leave your lungs.
7. Mindfulness is looking at the food you are about to prepare and wonder what the weather and soil conditions were like as it grew and how many hands it took to get that food to the table.

Mindfulness Images

- Imagine your consciousness connections.
- Imagine a sense of enlightenment, knowing you are part of all creation.
- Imagine the atoms passing through your body.
- Imagine you as billions of molecules spinning in space.
- Imagine everything in the universe is energy.
- Imagine IC is just energy changing form and leaving your body.

IC Imagery 12
Discomfort and Its Management
Supporting Health or Supporting Illness is the Game-Changer

There are two ways to look at the discomfort; both are game-changers. The body is calling out for help; you pay loving attention and take actions for soothing and comfort, or you curse the body, the discomfort, and beat yourself up with anger, distrust, negative self-talk, dread and worry, all increasing the discomfort.

1. You can obtain symptomatic relief and true physiologic healing depending on your imagination's response to the diagnosis, physician and treatment.
2. The imagination is like a wide open window or door, providing access to the power of the unconscious.
3. The unconscious mind can powerfully stimulate the healing response.
4. This response can in turn support tolerance with discomfort, necessary medical procedures and even the new normal.
5. Scientists have proven that positive imagery stimulates endorphins and valium, naturally occurring pain relieving substances in the central nervous system.

23

Managing Pain

Aristotle was the first to suggest "pain is an emotion" as pervasive as anger, terror, or joy. The emotional component of pain is bound to the physical experience of pain, creating anxiety, depression, agitation and a host of many other conditions. When you have hope, you can change your biology for healing. When you have hope, the body has a new normal response.

- Imagine your body healing in detail.
- Imagine feeling the bladder is comfortable, normal with healthy function.
- Imagine feeling happy with your support teams, the village of healers.
- Imagine you are sitting at a desk.
- On top of the desk is a pain meter with levels from 10 down to 1, then 0.
- Imagine turning down the pain meter.
- Make it real in your mind's eye and notice different sensations as you become more comfortable.

IC Imagery 13
Referred Pain
"Alice, please join the party,"
said the Mad Hatter

Referred pain is pain originating in the bladder
that is sometimes experienced in the sacrum,
tailbone, inner thigh, perineum, lower abdomen,
mid-back, bone structure, spine, fascia (holds the
bladder like an envelope), skin on the lower
abdomen and inner thighs.

1. Tight pelvic floor muscles irritate nerves,
    causing trigger points of pain along the
    length of the nerve and nerve endings and
    those nerves affect other places in the
    body.
2. Urgency with IC is the same feeling I
    remembered as a child when I played
    until the last minute, holding my legs
    together real tight, trying to not urinate
    on the way to the bathroom.
3. Urgency with IC is that same intense
    feeling multiple times, day and night.

What is Really Happening

- The purpose of the bladder's disconnect signal is to hold in the urine. The irritated bladder feels the need to release urine even when there is no urine.
- The pelvic floor muscles and the referred pain in other parts of the body all join the party to shut off the bladder. The very interesting fact is that the disconnect signal thinks its purpose is helping you.
- You can't be mad at the signal; however, you can consciously retrain the signal.

Helpful Images

- Imagine the bladder receiving the proper signals.
- Imagine the body relaxing and releasing all tensions.
- Imagine the tail bone, spine, lower and mid-back releasing all tension.
- Imagine the perineum cooling and softening.
- Imagine the skin returning to normal and loving to be touched.

IC Imagery 14
Dealing with Setbacks
Life is Always Full of Surprises and Unexpected Events

When you are doing everything right, moving ahead in your healing and then experience a setback, perhaps something else hurts or the burning returns or you have a flare-up, you may think, "Why me and why now?" The disappointment is sometimes overwhelming.

1. Symptoms are the body's way to heal itself or prevent further injury.
2. The wisdom of the nervous system easily motivates you to correct the situation.
3. You can change your reactions and adapt to ever-shifting demands during daily expected and unexpected events.
4. Examining the meaning of setback symptoms in a nonjudgmental way may give you deep insight; for example, if the body had a major flare-up right after an argument with someone. You can connect the flare-up with the stress and make changes accordingly.
5. With a treatment plan in place you will get through any setback; the symptoms will decrease, ultimately disappear and healing will happen.

Images to Help with Setbacks

- Imagine your knowledge as power.
- Imagine your power as healing.
- Imagine you are powerful beyond measure.
- Imagine using your wisdom to overcome setbacks.
- Imagine your life is returning to normal.

IC Imagery 15
Imagery and Physical Therapy
This is a Powerful Time for Your Body to Eavesdrop on Your Conversations

According to Albert Einstein, the words light and energy are the same and can be used interchangeably. Use this concept as part of your PT.

1. During your travel to the physical therapy (PT) clinic, before you arrive, imagine the clinic is filled with light and the energy of healing.
2. The clinic becomes a sacred space, holding all the prayers offered by each patient and therapist over many years.
3. Upon arrival at the clinic, take a brief moment, go within yourself and feel gratitude for the hands of light that are preparing for your treatment.
4. You are met with a welcoming warm smile, taken to the treatment room, given a gown and soon you are ready.
5. The Physical Therapist enters the room with a smile and encouragement and asks you what may have changed and what is happening in the body for today's adjustments.

Images for Physical Therapy Treatment

As the physical therapy treatment begins:

- Imagine you are connecting with the hands of light that are touching you.
- Imagine each fingertip is like a laser of directed energy.
- Imagine the intentions of your therapist and yourself working together with quantum mechanics and sending out thoughts of healing as a particle or a wave into the field of all possibility.
- Imagine the body relaxing as light enters each tight place, one by one.
- Imagine calming the nervous system just by breathing and allowing the wisdom of the treatment.
- Imagine the urethra, bladder and bladder lining as a channel for light energy.
- Imagine the cooling light soothing the connective tissue and muscles that are holding the bladder in place.
- Imagine being grateful for your body right now, as it is, with no judgment.

You've finished. Before you go…

Tweet/share that you finished this book.

Please star rate this book.

Reviews are solid gold to writers. Please
take a few minutes to give us some itty
bitty feedback.

ABOUT THE AUTHOR

Rhona first experienced Guided Imagery and Clinical Hypnosis when she was scheduled for a serious cancer surgery. The imagery was powerful and Rhona breezed through the procedure and recovered ahead of schedule. This life-changing event motivated Rhona to learn more about these powerful techniques.

An avid believer in the power of meditation, Rhona is a graduate of Chopra University, where she qualified as a Global Primordial Sound Meditation Instructor for the Chopra Center for Wellbeing. Rhona is also a certified Guided Imagery Therapist and Medical Hypnosis Instructor.

Rhona currently works from six clinics in Orange County, California, offering imagery and hypnosis to patients for pelvic floor dysfunction. She also maintains her private imagery and clinical hypnosis practice.

Rhona has been honored with a Humanitarian of the Year award in recognition of her work with trauma victims and first responders for the Trauma Intervention Program. She is also a sought-after motivational speaker. You can reach her at her website: www.rhonaimagery.com or by email at: Rhonaimagery@aol.com

Imagine what can be achieved!

Other Amazing Itty Bitty® Books

- **Your Amazing Itty Bitty® Imagery Book**
  – Rhona Jordan, C.GIt., C.CHt.

- **Your Amazing Itty Bitty® Meditation Book**
  – Rhona Jordan, C.GIt., C.CHt.

- **Your Amazing Itty Bitty® Bullying Book**
  – Colleen Monahan and Rhona Jordan, C.GIt., C.CHt.

- **Your Amazing Itty Bitty® Affirmations Book** - Micaela Passeri

With many more Amazing Itty Bitty® books available online…

Lightning Source UK Ltd.
Milton Keynes UK
UKHW021833290319
340174UK00025B/332/P

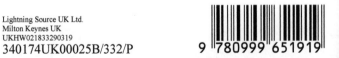